OUR EARTH JOURNEY

A HEALING NOTEBOOK BY JOY GARDNER

The Crossing P
Freedom, California 95019

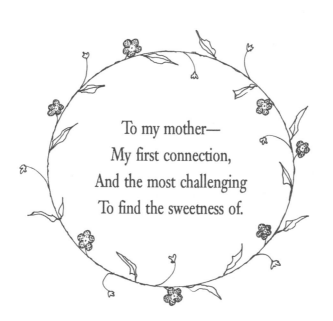

To my mother—
My first connection,
And the most challenging
To find the sweetness of.

Now the bird chirps.
Now the wind blows.
Fast. Then slow.
The willow bends in the wind;
the poplar trembles,
the brown-eyed Susans
speak amongst themselves—
all in vibrant harmony
with each other.

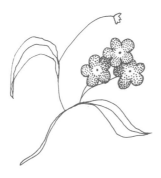

That is how it is with this book:
one page is the bird and another the willow;
you are the wind blowing through its pages.
Sometimes fast. Sometimes slow.

When we open to healing, all our relations will be there to help us: the trees, the birds, the flowers, the crystals—they will sing to us and welcome us back into the Family of Life. And we will remember that we are in the Garden of Eden.

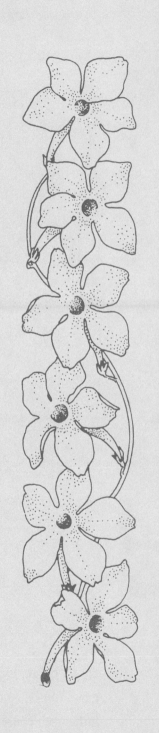

There are those who like to believe they have dominion over all the "lesser" kingdoms—yet in some sense, the opposite is true. No other life form has such a delicate, unstable, easily influenced energy field. Every life form that interacts with us leaves its mark upon us.

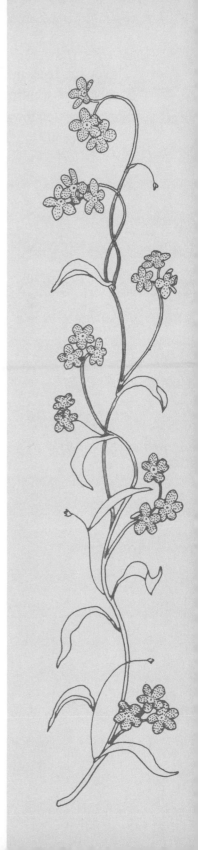

If you can rediscover your own unarmored child; if you can embrace your nurturing Earth Mother, then you will be taking one giant step toward healing yourself and healing the damage that unfeeling humans have brought upon this sweet planet.

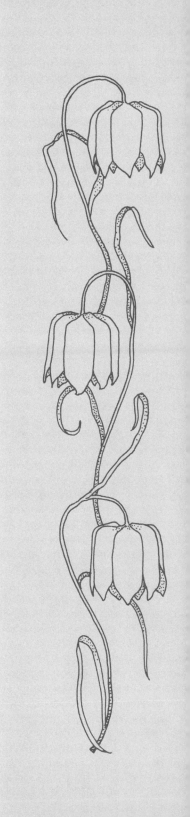

Go outdoors and attune to a particular tree, plant or flower. Drift back to when you were three or five or eight, when your backyard was a vast universe, and you were totally in love with the trees, the grass, the fairies.

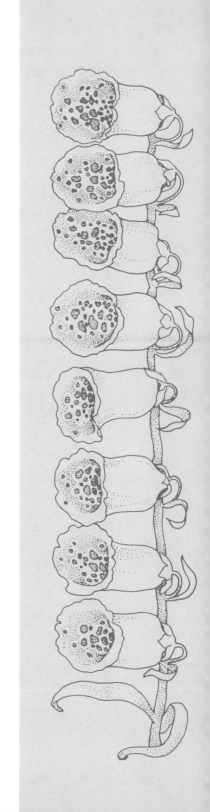

The Chinese symbol for man (human) is the same as for tree. Ancient Ones taught that humans are like trees because we have our roots in the earth and our heads in the heavens.

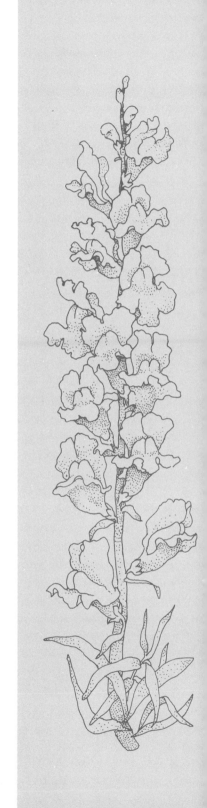

I have always loved trees. When I was little, I marveled that other people did not stare into the trees, watching the light reflecting off their leaves, watching their branches stir to and fro like great, loving arms.

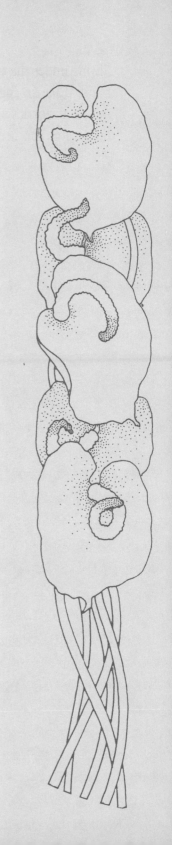

Sitting under the cedar tree, I feel its depth. It soothes my mind. Like an angel's wings, it spreads its fronds, sweeping away my worries and concerns, encouraging me to spread my own wings and become all that I can be.

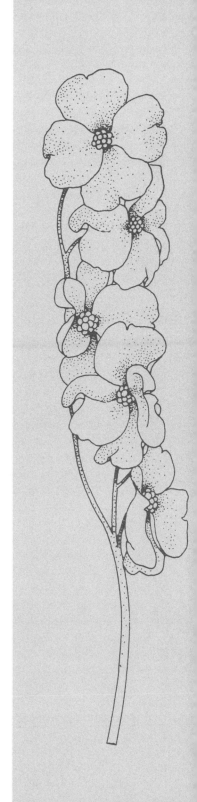

Pine is a purifier. Lie under a pine tree and notice the long sharp needles growing in clumps, dusting the air, constantly driving away negativity and dark energies, allowing in only the purest energy, the purest light. When we are in a pine forest, the aura receives a wondrous house-cleaning, even if we are entirely oblivious to the process.

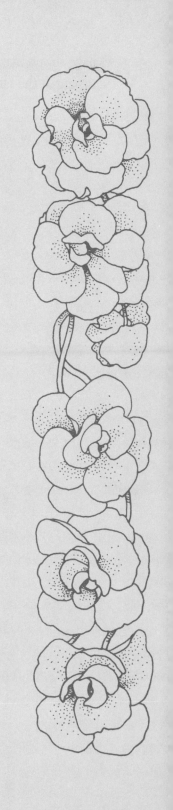

I have always marveled at how hundreds of birds can be chirping at the same time, and it sounds harmonious.

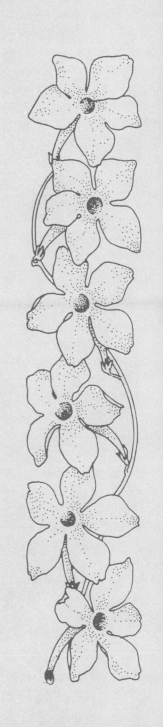

One way to find your gift is to consider the things you most enjoyed doing when you were a child. This will give you clues about your natural inclinations. You are "supposed" to do what you most deeply desire to do.

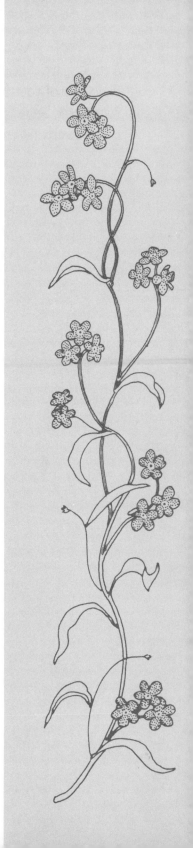

A major part of healing is to mend your heart. Your heart is at the center of your body and, when your heart energy flows, your whole being is full. Then you radiate love energy to everyone around you.

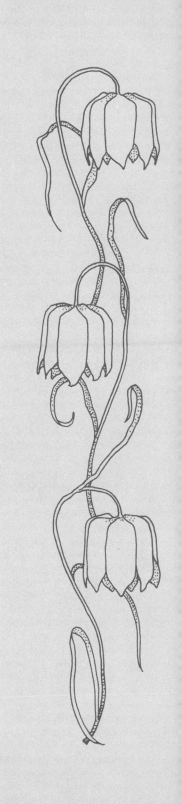

The honeycomb is the most secure structure. Every cell is open at either end, so that the sweetness can flow in and flow out. That's the only security there is. Try to give up all your constructs of how a relationship has to work.

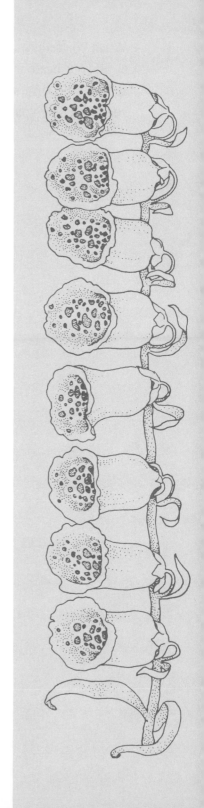

When you're hurt in life and love, the first impulse is to close down your heart and say, "I'll never let anyone do that to me again." Of course, when you build a wall around your heart, you're keeping yourself locked in.

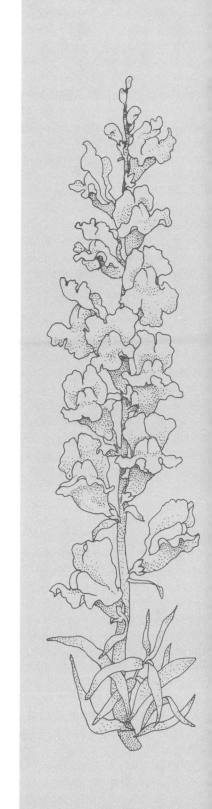

A short relationship can be a successful relationship. Just because it ended doesn't mean it failed. Each relationship is an opportunity for growth. All your previous relationships are the groundwork on which you build your present and future relationships.

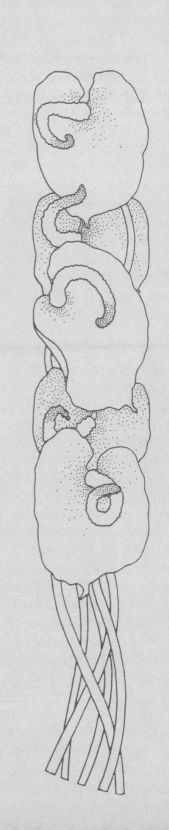

Sometimes you have to make a choice about whether to go forward into a new relationship that invariably falls short of your fantasies, or to go backward into the old life of security and fantasy, which can be infinitely delicious but entirely unsubstantial.

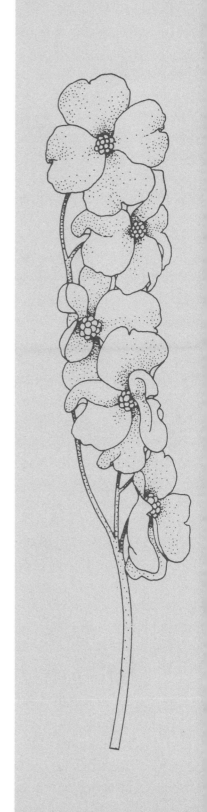

You can have a successful relationship as long as both of you are willing to change. Your partner is the one who knows you best; the one whom you have chosen as your mirror. So pay attention to each other. When you can both surrender to the needs of your partner, to the needs of the relationship, without being too uncomfortable, then you will be ready for intimacy.

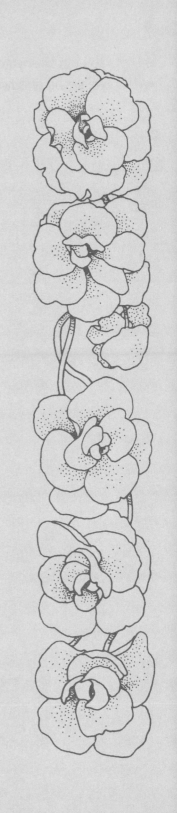

You can trust your partner when you feel confident that your vulnerability is not going to be used against you.

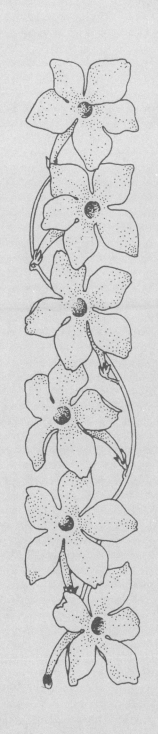

It's so precious when your partner really listens to you without being defensive. Then you feel heard; you feel cared for.

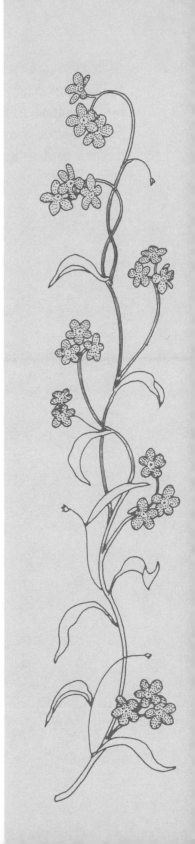

When you love each other as you are, change can occur willingly, gracefully, joyfully. Otherwise, resistance to change will be grating, painful, stubborn and resentful. Think of your relationship as a mutual adventure in tearing down armor, and become partners in this. Not adversaries, but partners.

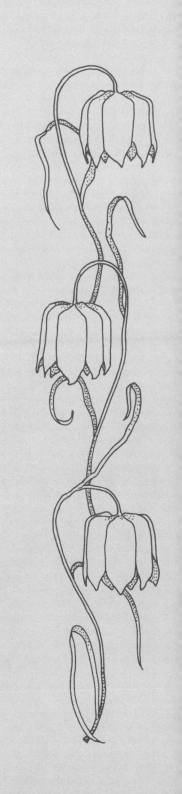

Women tend to carry their loyalty to their mothers into their relationships. Before you look at your mate through your mother's critical eyes, ask yourself whether *she* had a fulfilling love relationship.

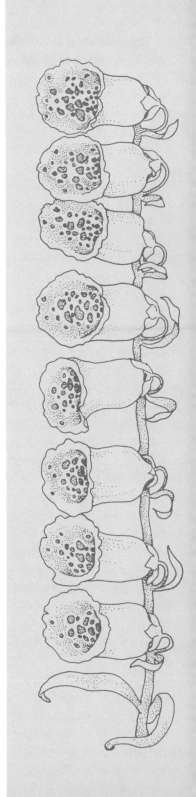

There's a controlling bitch in every woman and a manipulator in every man (or vice versa). Don't be afraid to admit it. You have to decide whether to be controlled by your monsters, or whether to take responsibility for them and calm them down.

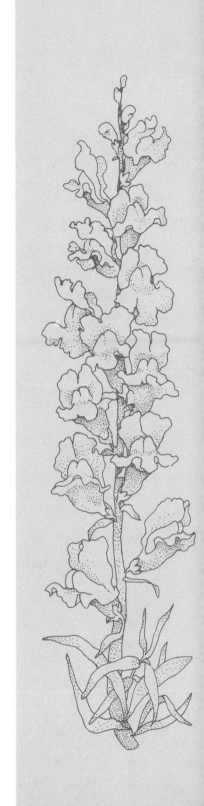

When you're the victim, no matter how people try to help you, they can't. So you're always in control. Because you can always be more of a victim than the other person can help you.

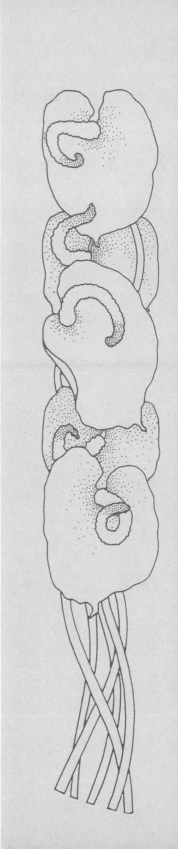

Watch out for the aspect of yourself that needs to be in control of everything and everyone in your environment. Having control over your partner (or your children) may make you feel secure, but it doesn't help to deepen your relationships.

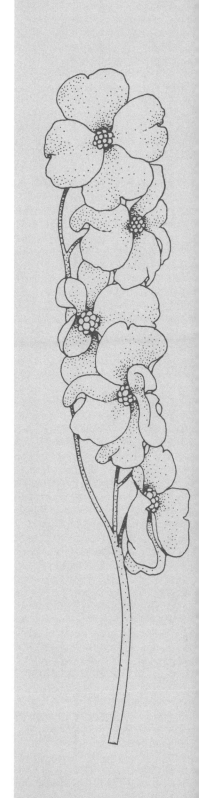

A loving relationship must be built on a foundation of self-acceptance and mutual acceptance. When you don't love yourself and you have no inner sense of what you really need, there's a tendency to set up laws and rules and rigid boundaries. When you're surrounded with fortresses, you can't open into an intimate relationship.

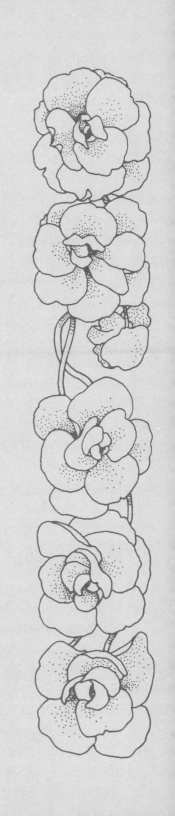

Fulfillment comes when we can take down the walls between who we are and who we pretend to be. We do this with each other by sharing our secrets, by daring to be vulnerable, by opening our hearts.

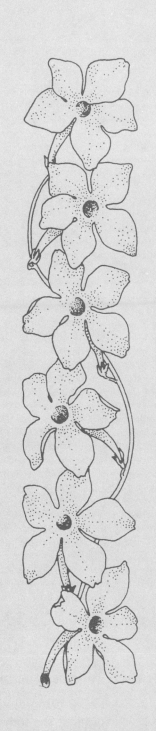

At some point, all the masks fall away: who you thought you were, who you thought you ought to be, who your parents wanted you to be. You let go and your True Self shines forth. No guilt, no need for illusion or pretense. "I am what I am."

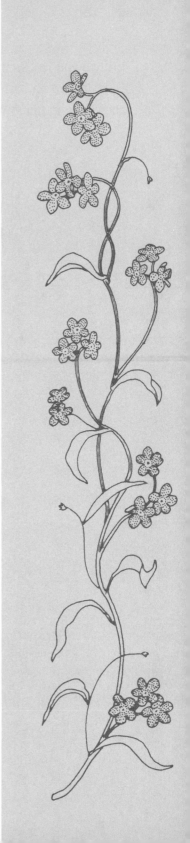

When you feel secure in your own identity, you can begin to give up certain parts of yourself in order to find yourself in a new way; in union with another.

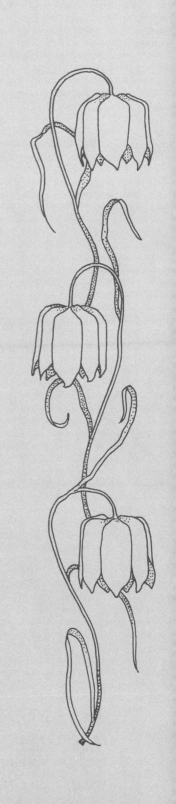

The goal is to be healed so that you no longer need each other in order to keep out of your misery. But if you sometimes feel needy, or if your partner feels needy, don't be afraid. This is who you are right now. Just relax and accept yourselves as you are.

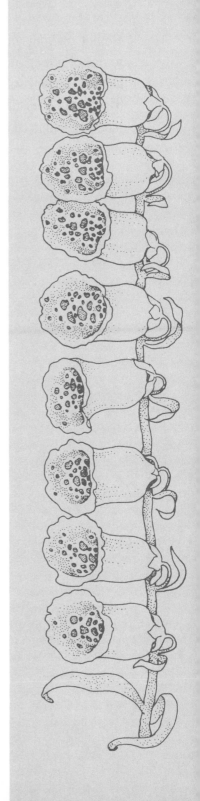

Do not cut yourself off from passion. It has its place. It is a source of power and self-confidence, which you should always have access to. Passion is an intensity of energy which is frightening or disturbing to many. But if you are to be whole, then you will need access to this part of your nature.

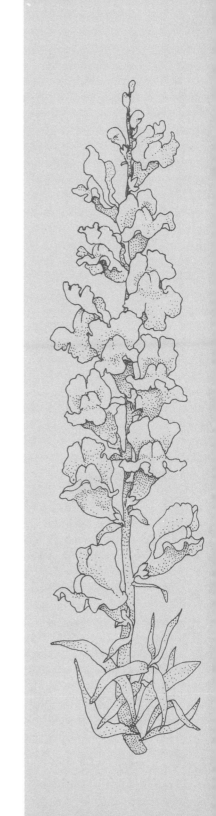

It's not sexual loyalty that's important. It's keeping the heart connection open. Sexual loyalty tends to go along with that. But people look at the symptom and think it's the root. Stay focused on the heart connection. Then everything else will take care of itself.

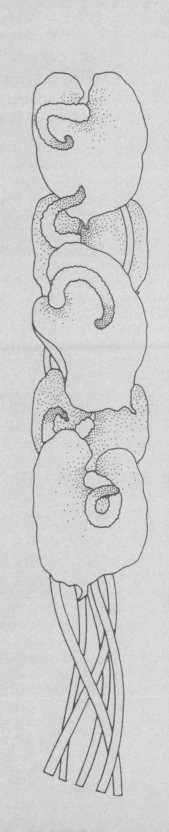

There's no commitment that two people can make that is as binding and exciting as choosing to have a baby together. It's miraculous when the love of two beings creates a third. It goes beyond any contractual agreement.

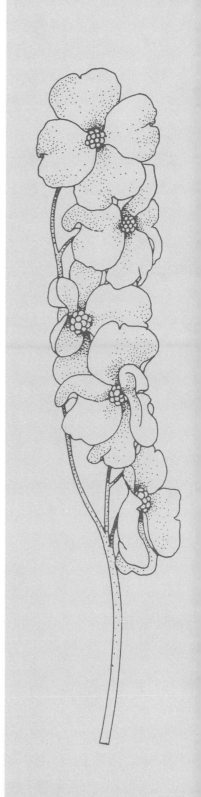

If you're considering having a baby and haven't found a partner, try to find someone you enjoy living with, because you'll be sharing your life with a child who closely resembles that person for a long, long time.

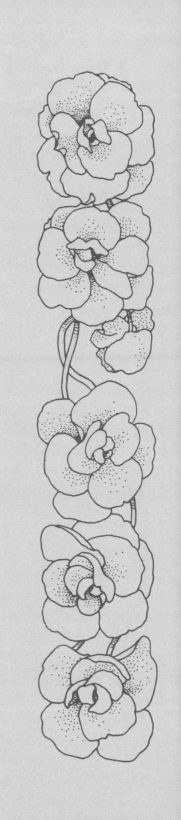

When a couple is in love, they glow. When they decide to have a baby, they share the miracle of knowing that their love can create a whole new being. When their seeds join, the radiance rises and you may know that they are pregnant just by looking at their faces.

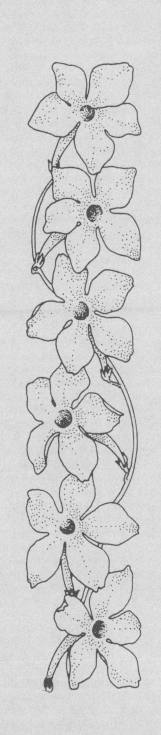

We tend to think that a baby in utero is entirely cut off from the world that lies just beyond a thin layer of skin. We seldom consider the child within as a conscious being, capable of responding to sound, emotions, and the inner environment that its mother creates through her sense of well-being, or lack of it.

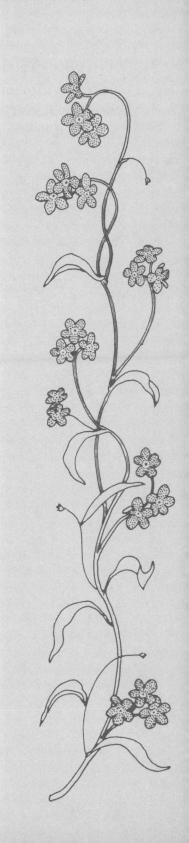

Research with plants shows that they like to be spoken to, they respond well to certain music, and grow more profusely when they're well loved and cared for. If this is true for a plant, it must be doubly true for the growing human baby.

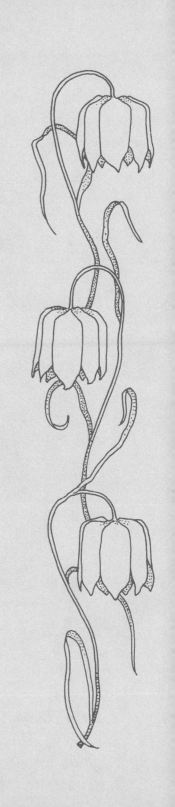

When a baby is inside its mother's belly, how does he or she feel loved? That growing baby can feel her love when she strokes her belly fondly, when she eats sensibly, when she talks and sings to her baby.

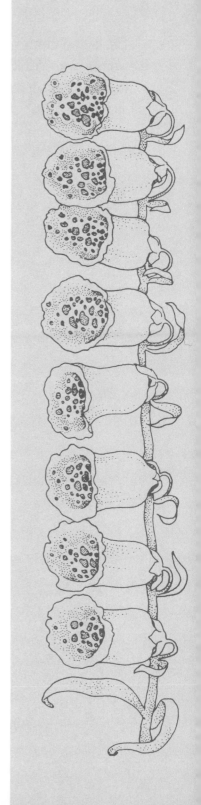

I've known many men who have ripened along with their women, who shared their partner's agonies and joys, who gave massages and support all through the delivery, and who love and nurture their children just as tenderly as any mother.

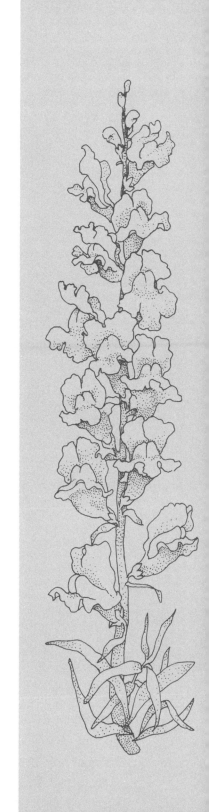

When fathers are given the opportunity to be alone with their newborns, they spend almost the same amount of time as mothers in holding, touching, and looking at these precious new creatures.

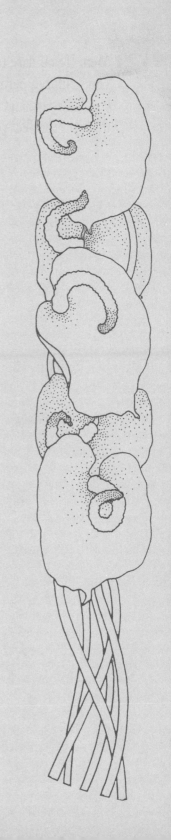

Men: If you dare to express your feelings, you will be giving your children permission to do so also. Children *need* to see you fall apart, and then pick up the pieces. They need to see that you can feel your feelings and still survive.

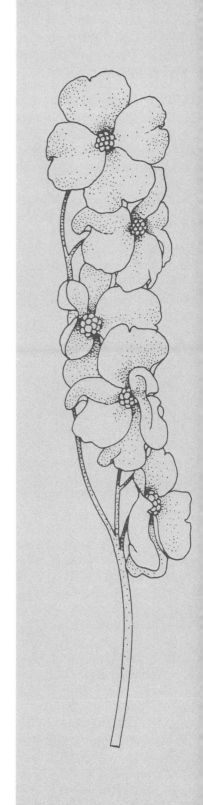

Eye-to-eye contact between mother and child during breast-feeding can be very rewarding. While you are nursing, the distance between your eyes and your infant's is the exact distance at which newborns can best focus.

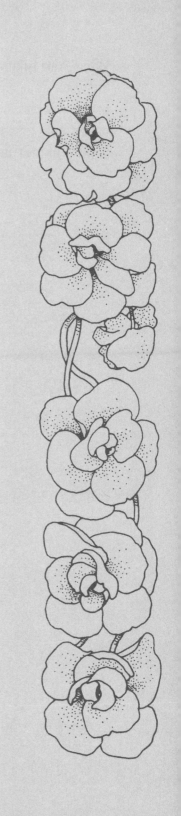

When your baby's eyes meet yours with complete trust, they have an openness which is virtually incomprehensible. In a baby's eyes, we see the miracle of life renewed—an opportunity for a part of ourselves to begin anew, without a backlog of pain and defensiveness.

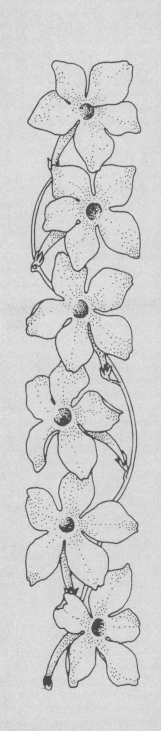

Seeing our newborn baby is literally falling
in love. It is the moment when we perceive that a part of
ourself, a part of our very flesh, is at one with Spirit. We see
ourselves in our baby's body, and we see pure spirit in our
baby's eyes. We smile at our baby, and Spirit smiles back at us.

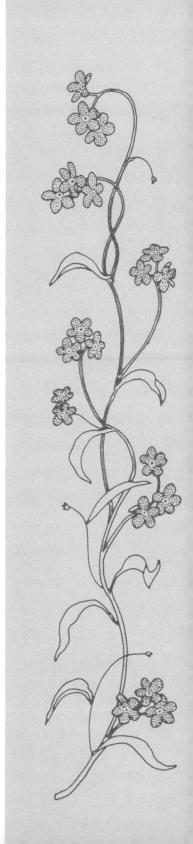

When parents or teachers have specific goals for children, this sets up a conflict in the child's will. The child will be torn between love for the parent or teacher, and the need to develop his or her own inner sense of knowingness.

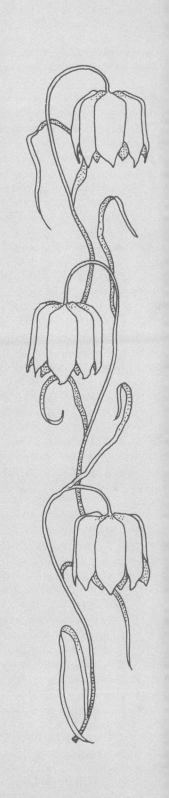

Holding a crystal is very much like holding a newborn baby. Being in the presence of a newborn's profound openness inspires us to reach deep inside ourselves and bring forth a complimentary openness.

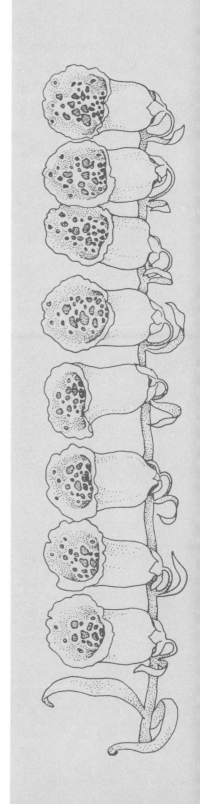

The crystals have been there all along, but we were blind to their beauty. Since they were so abundant, we didn't consider them precious. Similarly, the Light of Spirit has been there all along, but we've been blind to it because we didn't love ourselves.

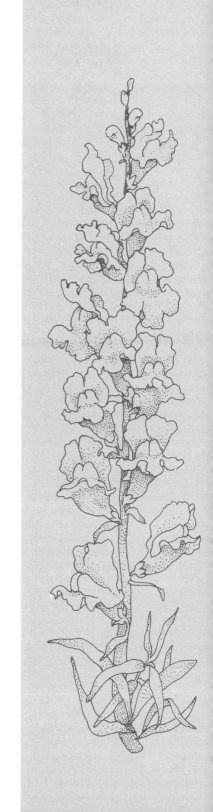

Now that we're moving toward the Light, the crystals are ready to reflect back the Light that we're finding within. The infinite variety of crystals assures us that we can be totally unique and remain beautifully in the Light.

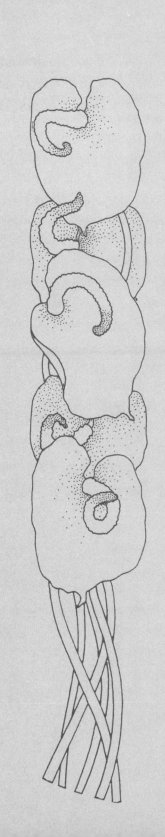

If you are drawn to a particular crystal, then you are in harmony with its energy, and you don't have to worry about whether it is chipped or not. We all have chips of one kind or another.

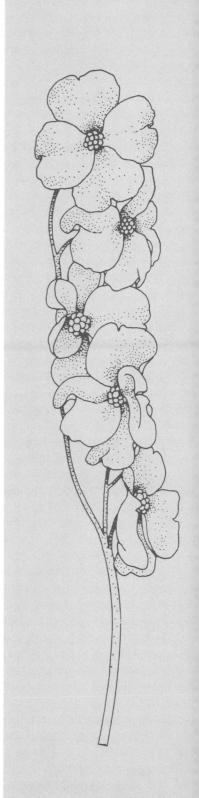

Smoky Quartz. Use this stone in a room where there are negative energies such as jealousy, resentment, or deliberate confusion. It will thicken those energies so that they become heavy and merge with the earth.

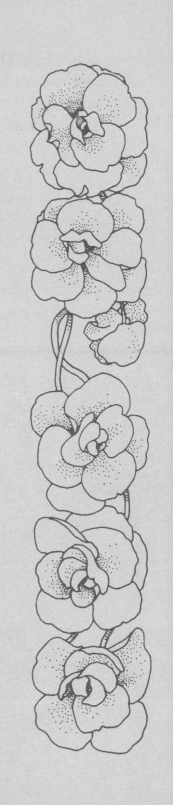

Tiger's Eye. This is a stone of courage. It gives strength and endurance and the willingness to go forward in spite of obstacles. By stroking its smooth surface you will soothe away your worries and apprehensions.

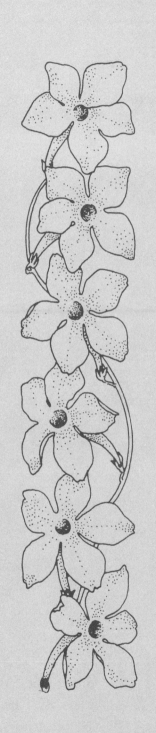

Green Jade. When your heart feels threatened or frightened, jade is like a loving father, reaching out his hand to give comfort, reassurance, and protection. It has a gentle strength, and it conveys that strength to the one who wears it.

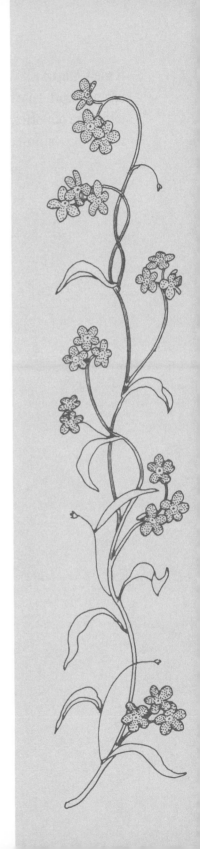

Rose Quartz. If you've been hurt in love or suffer from a broken heart, rose quartz is like the Divine Mother, the ultimate comforter, who rocks you in her arms and gives you unconditional love.

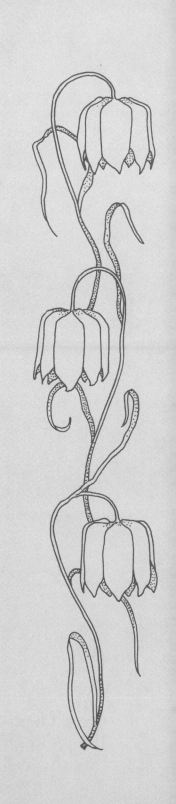

Crystal Cluster. The cluster is the perfect group crystal. Here you see a multitude of unique, powerful individuals, each going off in a separate direction, yet joined at the base, the stone matrix from which they all emerge.

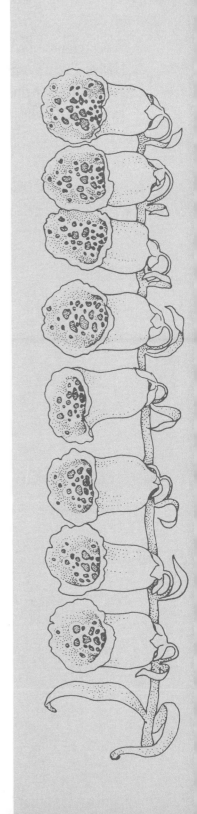

When groups of people gather together and align with a Higher Consciousness, then a great power is available. This group, however small, has access to Divine forces, and can have a great influence on planetary energies.

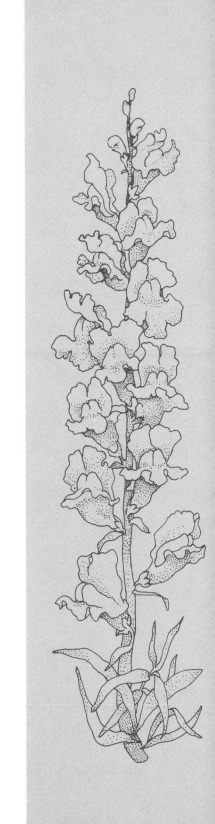

If you belong to a group that has a higher purpose, find a crystal cluster that reflects the perfection of your group. Place it at the center of the room, or at the center of your meditation circle when you gather. It will help your group attune to the higher powers and to its own perfection.

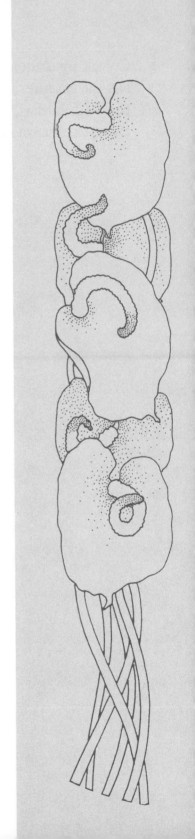

Crystals are like teachers. True teachers embody their teachings and emanate those teachings through their eyes and every pore of their being, so that even if they never say a word, you can receive that knowledge simply by being in their presence.

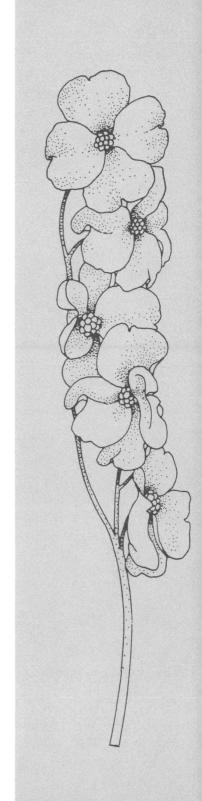

A teacher is a person who—in some sense—I want to be like. When I am near this person, I absorb some part of their essence, through a kind of osmosis. The Hopi Indians never 'taught' me anything. But once they decided they could trust me, they allowed me to be in their presence. And that was everything.

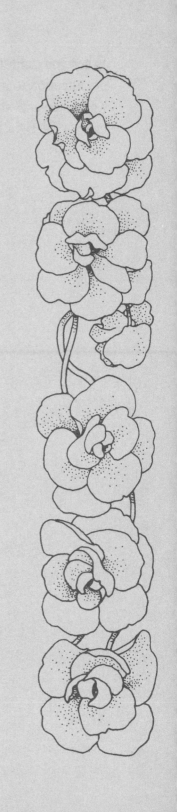

When you can listen to your intuition, your inner voice, and pay attention to it, your life will change. You will always know what to do and when to do it. You will always be at the right place at the right time.

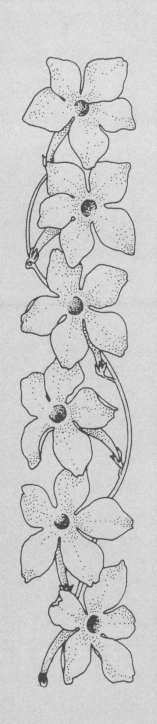

The way we come into this life and the way we depart from it set the tone for this life and the life beyond.

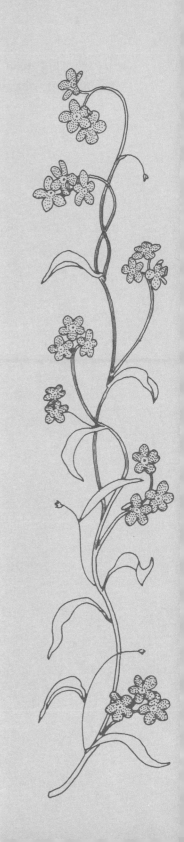

By releasing anger and sorrow from the past, we stand fully in the present, vibrating, full of life and joy.

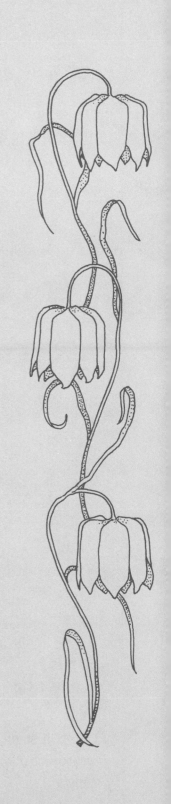

The greatest gift that one human being can give another is unconditional love. It's the only thing, ultimately, that really matters.

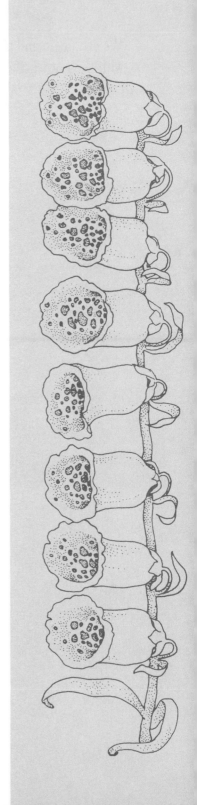

We can begin and end our lives in harmony with ourselves, with each other, the plants, the animals, the earth, and the cosmos.

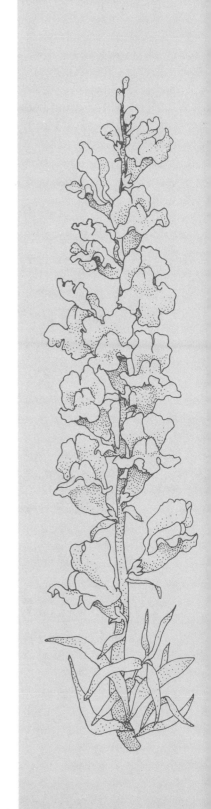

The following books by Joy Gardner are published by
The Crossing Press:

Color and Crystals, A Journey Through the Chakras
The New Healing Yourself, Natural Remedies for Adults and Children
Healing Yourself During Pregnancy
A Difficult Decision, A Compassionate Book about Abortion

Also published by The Crossing Press are these gift journals:

A Women's Notebook
A Women's Book
Water Spirit
Moon Spirit
Moon Flower
A Journal for Cat Lovers
The Goddess Remembered
Earth Songs

To receive a current catalog of books published by
The Crossing Press, please call—Toll Free—800/777/1048.